CHAIR YOGA FOR

SENIORS AND

BEGINNERS

Learn to practice Chair Yoga for Seniors or people with reduced mobility with this guide.

Dorothy Snow

CONTENTS

I

Introduction

Chair yoga, an adapted and gentle yoga practice, has become a transformative choice for seniors aiming for holistic well-being. Different from traditional yoga, chair yoga modifies poses to be done while seated, offering an inclusive exercise option suitable for individuals with varying levels of mobility. This adaptation enables seniors to experience the physical and mental benefits of yoga without requiring complex movements or intense physical effort.

The importance of physical activity grows substantially as individuals age. Sustaining an active lifestyle becomes increasingly vital for overall health. Regular exercise not only enhances physical strength and flexibility but also plays a pivotal role in reducing the risk of chronic conditions like cardiovascular diseases and osteoporosis. Beyond the physical benefits, regular exercise positively impacts mental well-being by alleviating stress, anxiety, and improving cognitive function.

The 90-day weight loss plan presented in this guide is tailored to meet the specific needs of seniors. The primary goals are diverse, aiming for not only weight loss but also overall enhancement in physical fitness, mental clarity, and emotional well-being. Through a blend of chair yoga routines, personalized nutritional guidance, and motivational support, the plan empowers seniors to embark on a transformative journey toward a healthier, more vibrant lifestyle.

Within this comprehensive framework, the objectives include gradual and sustainable weight loss, the development of strength and flexibility, the establishment of positive dietary habits, and the cultivation of a sense of accomplishment and confidence. The 90-day timeline is strategic, offering a structured yet adaptable approach, allowing seniors to progress at their own pace and ensuring that the journey towards weight loss is both enjoyable and achievable.

Embracing the chair yoga for seniors' 90-day weight loss plan means investing not only in physical health but also in establishing the groundwork for a more fulfilling and active senior life. This introduction sets the stage for an exploration of chair yoga's transformative potential and the positive impact it can have on the lives of seniors seeking a holistic approach to weight loss and overall well-being.

II

Getting Started with Chair Yoga

Advantages of Yoga for Senior

1.) Enhances Mental Acuity: Engaging in yoga fosters a calm and reflective atmosphere, slowing down breathing and encouraging meditation. This practice promotes mental sharpness and cognitive function, offering a respite from the fast-paced nature of daily life and fostering improved mood and memory.

2.) Strengthens Bones and Joints: As aging progresses, bones lose density, and joints become stiffer, potentially leading to issues like osteoporosis. Gentle yoga proves effective in preventing or slowing the loss of bone density, alleviating joint and bone pain, and is considered safe for those with osteoporosis. Regular joint movement can reduce stiffness and tenderness.

3.) Boosts Balance and Stamina: The deliberate and measured movements in yoga, coupled with pose-holding, contribute to improved balance and increased strength with age. Despite initial wobbliness, consistent yoga practice gradually enhances the ability to perform poses and maintain balance.

4.) Easing stress: Participating in yoga classes proves highly effective in alleviating stress and tension, potentially leading to a reduction in required medication. Researchers suggest that yoga's combination of postures, meditation, and controlled breathing may decrease nervous system activity, aiding in the management of blood pressure.

5.) Enhancing sleep quality: Many individuals note improved sleep and reduced insomnia upon incorporating yoga into their routine. Engaging in simple stretches or breathing exercises before bedtime promotes mindfulness, shifting focus from daily concerns to the present moment.

6.) Slowing the aging process: The fundamental tenets of yoga, namely strength and relaxation, play pivotal roles in decelerating the aging process. Yoga's calming effect on breathing enhances circulation and lowers heart rate, while strength-building counters age-related muscle loss, potentially even reversing it.

7.) Alleviating back pain: Yoga is instrumental in bolstering back strength, flexibility, and core stability, addressing posture issues and fostering healthy breathing practices—essential components for maintaining a strong back. It stands out as an effective tool in reducing lower back pain, a prevalent source of discomfort and disability among older adults.

NOTE: *Yoga postures aim to enhance muscle flexibility and strength without causing pain. It is crucial never to push oneself to the point of discomfort. Communicate any physical issues or pain to your yoga instructor for appropriate adjustments to your routine and sequence.*

Basic Chair Yoga Poses

Chair yoga, tailored for accessibility and ease, introduces a range of foundational poses that foster physical well-being and mindfulness.

These poses, adapted for seated or chair-supported practice, establish a gentle yet impactful exercise routine suitable for seniors. Let's delve into the nuances of key chair yoga poses:

1. Seated Mountain Pose:

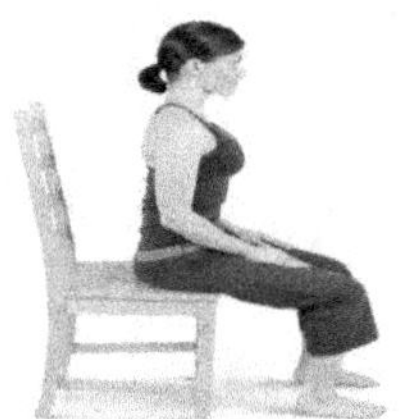

✔ Sit comfortably, ensuring a straight back

and feet flat on the floor.

✔ Inhale, lifting your arms overhead with palms facing each other.

✔ Engage your core, promoting spine elongation.

✔ Maintain a steady and comfortable breathing pattern.

This pose cultivates better posture, spine flexibility, and heightened body awareness.

2. Chair Cat-Cow Stretch:

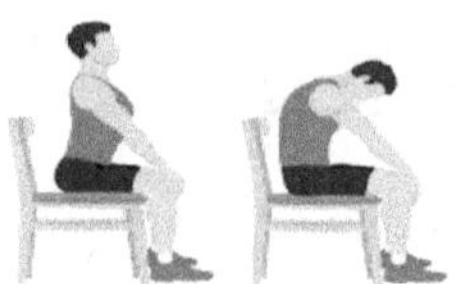

✔ Sit at the chair's edge with hands resting

on your knees.

✔ Inhale, arching your back and raising your

chest (Cow).

✔ Exhale, rounding your spine, bringing

your chin to your chest (Cat).

Repeat this seamless motion to enhance spinal flexibility and alleviate back tension.

3. Seated Forward Bend:

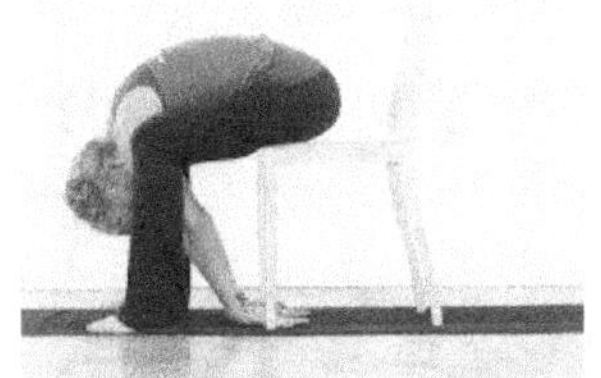

✔ Sit with feet hip-width apart, firmly grounded.

✔ Inhale, lengthening your spine; exhale, hinging at the hips and reaching forward.

✔ Extend arms toward the floor, feeling a

gentle stretch in the lower back and

hamstrings.

✔ Adjust the stretch intensity according to

your comfort.

4. Seated Twist:

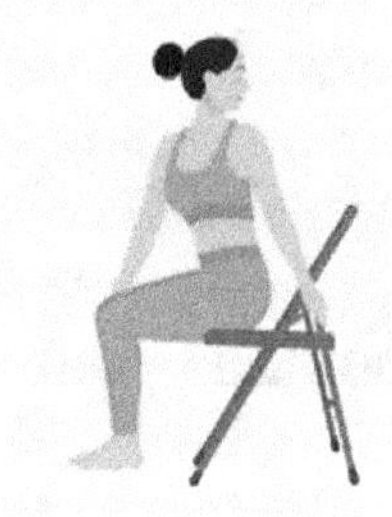

✔ Sit tall with feet flat on the floor.

✔ Inhale, lengthen your spine; exhale, twist your upper body to one side.

✔ Place one hand on the opposite knee and the other on the chair's back.

✔ Hold the twist, alternating sides.

This pose enhances spinal mobility and supports a mild detoxification effect.

5. Chair Warrior Pose:

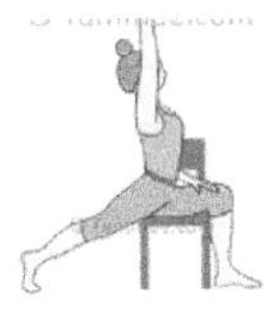

✔ Sit with wide-set feet and toes slightly outward.

✔ Inhale, lift your arms to shoulder height, palms facing down.

✔ Exhale, bend your right knee, lowering the right arm for a side stretch.

✔ Inhale back to centre; exhale to the other side.

This modified Warrior Pose strengthens the legs and enhances balance.

6. Chair Tree Pose:

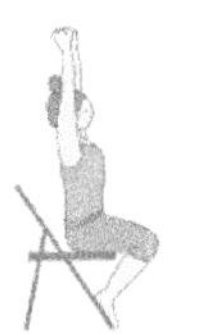

✔ Sit tall, feet flat on the floor.

✔ Lift your right foot, placing the sole

against the inner left thigh or calf.

✔ Palms together in front of your chest.

✔ Hold, focusing on a point for balance;

switch sides.

Chair Tree Pose hones balance and concentration.

Mastery of these foundational chair yoga poses establishes the groundwork for a rewarding and beneficial practice. As seniors become acquainted with these gentle movements, they can confidently progress toward enhanced flexibility, balance, and overall well-being. The adaptable nature of these poses ensures individuals of all fitness levels can embrace the transformative essence of chair yoga with ease and assurance.

Safety Measures for Seniors in Chair Yoga

Ensuring the well-being of seniors during chair yoga involves meticulous attention to specific safety measures. These precautions are designed to establish a secure and enjoyable setting, catering to individuals with diverse mobility levels and health considerations.

1. Selecting a Solid Chair: Choose a chair that is stable and positioned on a non-slip surface to minimize the risk of unintended slips or falls.

2. Avoiding Unstable Chairs: Discourage the use of chairs with wheels or excessive

height, as these may compromise stability during poses.

3. Promoting Mindfulness: Advocate for mindfulness during chair yoga, prompting seniors to be attuned to their bodies and movements to prevent overexertion or strain.

4. Attending to Body Signals: Stress the significance of heeding their bodies, allowing for modifications or breaks to avert discomfort or potential injury.

5. Consultation with Healthcare Professionals: Encourage seniors to consult with healthcare professionals

before commencing chair yoga, particularly if they have existing health conditions or concerns.

6. Acknowledging Medical Histories: Inquire about participants' medical histories to customize the practice, accommodating any specific health considerations or limitations.

7. Ensuring Safe Poses: Emphasize the necessity of maintaining proper alignment during poses to prevent strain on joints and muscles.

8. Providing Clear Instructions: Deliver clear and succinct instructions, ensuring

participants comprehend correct posture and movements to minimize the risk of injury.

9. Structured Advancement: Organize chair yoga sessions to commence with simpler poses and gradually progress to more intricate ones, allowing seniors to adapt to the practice at their own pace.

10. Adjustable Intensity: Grant participants control over the intensity of their practice, underlining that progress is a gradual and individualized process.

11. Encouraging Open Communication: Foster transparent communication

between seniors and instructors, urging participants to express any discomfort or concerns during the session.

12. Offering Personalized Support: Provide tailored assistance and modifications, recognizing the unique needs and capabilities of each participant.

13. Incorporating Props Judiciously: Integrate props like blocks or cushions thoughtfully to offer additional support and enrich the yoga experience.

14. Educating on Prop Usage: Educate participants on the correct usage of props,

ensuring they understand how to integrate them safely into their practice.

Implementing these safety measures establishes an environment where seniors can confidently participate in chair yoga, knowing that their safety and comfort are prioritized. Through a blend of awareness, clear communication, and personalized attention, chair yoga sessions become not just physically beneficial but emotionally reassuring for seniors on their wellness journey.

Customizing Routines to Fitness Levels

Customizing chair yoga routines for seniors is crucial to make the practice inclusive and effective, considering diverse fitness levels. This personalized approach empowers individuals to engage in a yoga experience that aligns with their abilities, fostering a positive and empowering atmosphere.

1. Pose Adaptation:

Offering Pose Variations: Provide a range of pose variations for participants to choose from, allowing them to select modifications that suit their fitness levels and comfort.

Flexibility in Approach: Emphasize the adaptable nature of chair yoga, allowing participants to progress from simpler to more advanced poses as their confidence and strength grow.

2. Gradual Advancement:

Structured Progression: Structure routines to begin with basic poses, gradually introducing more challenging ones. This approach helps participants build strength and flexibility over time.

Personalized Pace: Encourage participants to move at their own pace, ensuring a comfortable practice and the ability to adjust the intensity as needed.

3. Personalized Guidance:

Open Communication: Establish clear communication channels to understand participants' fitness levels, preferences, and any concerns.

Individual Support: Provide personalized guidance during sessions, offering modifications or extra support based on each participant's specific needs.

4. Use of Props:

Prop Inclusion: Introduce props such as straps, blocks, or cushions to assist and enhance poses.

Educational Focus: Educate participants on the role of props, emphasizing their contribution to making the practice accessible to individuals with diverse fitness levels.

5. Encouraging Self-Assessment:

Promoting Body Awareness: Encourage self-awareness, prompting participants to assess their comfort levels during poses.

Empowering Choices: Empower participants by highlighting that modifying or skipping poses is a valid choice to ensure a safe and enjoyable practice.

6. Flexible Duration:

Shorter Sessions: Acknowledge that some participants may prefer shorter sessions initially. Provide options for gradually extending practice durations as participants become more accustomed to chair yoga.

Adaptable Commitment: Allow participants to customize the frequency of their practice, recognizing that consistency is more important than duration.

7. Emphasis on Breath and Mindfulness:

Universal Focus: Regardless of fitness level, stress the significance of breath and mindfulness in chair yoga.

Accessible Mindfulness Practices: Introduce mindfulness techniques that seamlessly integrate into routines, promoting a holistic well-being approach.

Tailoring chair yoga routines to fitness levels ensures inclusivity and empowers seniors to embrace a practice that suits their unique capabilities. By emphasizing adaptability, gradual progression, and individualized support,

chair yoga becomes an accessible and versatile

avenue for seniors to enhance both their

physical and mental well-being.

III

Nutrition Guide for Seniors

Maintaining optimal health in the senior years' hinges on sound nutritional choices. This section delves into the significance of a well-rounded diet, emphasizes nutrient-packed foods conducive to weight loss, and navigates dietary nuances tailored to the specific needs of seniors.

Significance of a Balanced Diet

Ensuring seniors receive a spectrum of essential nutrients is pivotal for their health and vitality.

The following facets underscore the importance of a balanced diet:

1. Nutrient Adequacy:

A balanced diet guarantees seniors receive essential vitamins, minerals, proteins, carbohydrates, and fats, sustaining immune function and overall well-being.

2. Energy Maintenance:

Caloric needs may shift with age, and a balanced diet aids in maintaining an appropriate energy balance, essential for daily activities and muscle preservation.

3. Disease Prevention:

A diet rich in fruits, vegetables, and whole grains offers antioxidants and fibre, thwarting chronic diseases like heart ailments and certain cancers.

4. Digestive Health:

Inclusion of fibre from diverse sources promotes digestive health, countering common issues like constipation prevalent among seniors.

5. Hydration:

Seniors face an elevated risk of dehydration, making sufficient fluid intake critical for cognitive function, joint health, and overall bodily functions.

Nutrient-Rich Foods for Weight Loss

For seniors aiming for weight loss, the focus shifts to nutrient-dense foods to support this goal healthily:

- Lean Proteins:

Lean protein sources such as fish, poultry, tofu, and legumes are chosen to preserve muscle mass while managing calorie intake.

- Colourful Vegetables:

A variety of colourful vegetables ensures a broad nutrient spectrum, with their low-calorie, high-fibre nature promoting satiety and aiding weight loss.

- Whole Grains:

Emphasis is placed on whole grains like quinoa and brown rice, providing increased fibre for sustained energy release.

- Healthy Fats:

Moderate inclusion of healthy fats from avocados, nuts, and olive oil supports nutrient absorption and satiety.

- Low-Fat Dairy:

Low-fat or fat-free dairy options are recommended to ensure sufficient calcium without excess saturated fats.

- Fruits as Sweeteners:

Fruits are utilized as natural sweeteners, reducing calorie intake while providing essential vitamins and antioxidants.

- Hydration with Water:

Water takes precedence as the main beverage to ensure hydration without unnecessary calorie consumption.

Dietary Considerations for Seniors

Seniors encounter specific dietary considerations tied to changes in metabolism, digestion, and nutrient absorption. Addressing these is paramount for their overall well-being:

- Caloric Needs:

Awareness that caloric needs may decrease with age necessitates adjustments to portion sizes to prevent excessive calorie intake.

- Protein Intake:

An emphasis on adequate protein intake supports muscle health, recognizing the potential for slightly higher protein requirements in seniors.

- Fibre for Digestive Health:

A priority is placed on fibre-rich foods to maintain digestive health, preventing constipation, and fostering a healthy gut microbiome.

- Calcium and Vitamin D:

Ensuring sufficient calcium and vitamin D intake is crucial for bone health and fracture risk reduction.

- Hydration Awareness:

Mindful hydration is encouraged, considering the diminished sense of thirst among seniors.

- Medical Conditions:

Tailoring dietary plans to existing medical conditions ensures a holistic approach, necessitating consultation with healthcare professionals for personalized recommendations.

- Nutrient-Dense Snacking:

Advocating for nutrient-dense snacks between meals maintains energy levels without compromising overall caloric goals.

- Meal Timing:

Considering meal timing aligns with seniors' daily routines, ensuring sustained energy throughout the day.

By embracing these principles, seniors can fortify their nutritional intake, bolster overall health, and embark on a journey toward sustained well-being in their golden years.

IV

90-Day Chair Yoga Weight Loss Plan

Embarking on a transformative journey toward weight loss through chair yoga necessitates a systematic and sustainable approach. This 90-day plan is intricately crafted to guide seniors through a series of chair yoga routines, with a focal point on a weekly breakdown, progressive intensity, and the pivotal role of tracking progress for efficacious and fulfilling outcomes.

Weekly Breakdown of Chair Yoga Routines

Weeks 1-2: Establishing Foundations and Familiarity

Days 1-3: Introduction to Seated Poses

Initiate with gentle poses like Seated Mountain, Chair Cat-Cow, and Seated Forward Bend to foster familiarity.

Emphasize proper breathing techniques and mindful awareness.

Days 4-7: Incorporating Mobility

Introduce Seated Twist and Gentle Chair Warrior Pose.

Focus on smooth transitions and sustaining comfortable postures.

Weeks 3-4: Cultivating Flexibility and Balance

Days 8-14: Expansion of Poses

Incorporate additional poses such as Seated Tree Pose and Seated Warrior.

Emphasize stretching for enhanced flexibility while seated.

Days 15-21: Sequenced Seated Flows

Integrate sequenced routines combining learned poses.

Encourage fluid movements to enhance balance and coordination.

Weeks 5-6: Strengthening Core and Lower Body

Days 22-28: Focus on Core Strength

Introduce core-focused poses like Seated Boat Pose and Leg Lifts.

Include gentle abdominal exercises while seated.

Days 29-35: Emphasis on Lower Body

Concentrate on poses such as Chair Squats and Leg Extensions.

Gradually progress to enhance lower body strength.

Weeks 7-8: Mastery of Advanced Seated Poses

Days 36-42: Exploration of Advanced Poses

Introduce challenging poses like Seated Camel Pose and Seated Pigeon.

Emphasize maintaining comfort and alignment in more intricate positions.

Days 43-49: Dynamic Seated Sequences

Incorporate dynamic sequences that combine advanced poses.

Encourage controlled movements for an advanced fitness experience.

Weeks 9-10: Integrating Full Body Movements

Days 50-56: Comprehensive Chair Yoga Sessions

Engage in full-length chair yoga sessions combining all learned poses.

Focus on flow, synchronization of breath, and maintaining a balanced practice.

Days 57-63: Interval Training with Chair Poses

Introduce interval training principles, incorporating chair poses.

Alternate between moderate and higher intensity for cardiovascular benefits.

Weeks 11-12: Culmination and Mastery

Days 64-77: Mastery of Chair Yoga Weight Loss Plan

Focus on refining techniques, holding poses with increased stability, and mastering seamless transitions.

Introduce customized routines based on individual preferences and strengths.

Days 78-90: Personalized Challenge and Integration

Encourage participants to personalize their chair yoga routine.

Gradually increase session duration and intensity for those ready to embrace additional challenges.

Gradual Intensity Progression
Phase 1: Gentle Introduction (Weeks 1-4)

Objective: Establish a foundation, foster familiarity with chair yoga, and promote consistent practice.

Intensity Level: Low to moderate.

Guidelines: Focus on gentle poses, controlled breathing, and mindfulness in movements.

Phase 2: Building Strength and Flexibility (Weeks 5-8)

Objective: Introduce more poses, enhance flexibility, and gradually increase the challenge.

Intensity Level: Moderate.

Guidelines: Incorporate a variety of poses targeting different muscle groups. Emphasize smooth transitions.

Phase 3: Advanced Poses and Sequences (Weeks 9-10)

Objective: Explore advanced seated poses and dynamic sequences for a holistic workout.

Intensity Level: Moderate to high.

Guidelines: Introduce challenging poses progressively. Focus on maintaining form and flow during sequences.

Phase 4: Full Body Integration and Interval Training (Weeks 11-12)

Objective: Integrate all learned poses, emphasize full-body engagement, and introduce interval training principles.

Intensity Level: High.

Guidelines: Combine sequences into longer sessions. Incorporate intervals for cardiovascular benefits.

Tracking Progress and Adjustments
Tracking Methods:

1. Daily Journaling: Participants are encouraged to maintain a daily journal, noting session duration, perceived effort, and any modifications made.

2. Photographic Progress: Regular photos can visually track changes in posture and flexibility.

3. Measurement Metrics: Tracking weight, body measurements, and overall well-being.

Progress Assessment:

1. Bi-weekly Check-Ins: Regular check-ins are scheduled to assess progress, discuss challenges, and provide personalized feedback.

2. Instructor Feedback: Open communication with the instructor is

maintained to address concerns and receive guidance on adjustments.

Adjustments and Customization:

1. Individualized Modifications: Acknowledge that progress varies; modifications can be made based on individual capabilities.

2. Flexible Program Structure: Allow participants to repeat certain weeks or modify routines as needed to accommodate changes in fitness levels or preferences.

3. Consultation with Healthcare Professionals: Encourage consultation

with healthcare professionals if discomfort or health-related concerns arise, enabling personalized adjustments.

Celebrating Milestones:

Recognition of Achievements: Small victories and milestones are celebrated during the 90-day journey.

Encouragement for Consistency: Participants are reminded of the importance of consistent practice and the positive impact of chair yoga on overall well-being.

This 90-day chair yoga weight loss plan offers a systematic approach to gradual progression, ensuring participants build strength, flexibility, and overall fitness. The emphasis on tracking progress and making personalized adjustments fosters a supportive environment, empowering seniors to achieve their weight loss goals through a sustainable and enriching chair yoga practice.

V

Motivational Tips for Seniors

Embarking on a journey toward health and well-being is a rewarding endeavour, especially for seniors. This section delves into motivational tips tailored for seniors, encompassing inspiring quotes and affirmations, setting achievable goals, and the significance of fostering a supportive community.

Encouraging Quotes and Affirmations

1. Affirmations for Positivity:

Quote: "Today, I choose joy and vitality. My age is a testament to my wisdom and resilience."

Affirmation: "I embrace each day with gratitude and strength, acknowledging the richness of my experiences."

2. Embracing Change:

Quote: "The only way to make sense out of change is to plunge into it, move with it, and join the dance." – Alan Watts

Affirmation: "I welcome change as an opportunity for growth, understanding that every step forward is a dance with life's rhythm."

3. Empowerment Through Challenges:

Quote: "It's not whether you get knocked down, it's whether you get up." – Vince Lombardi

Affirmation: "Challenges are stepping stones to my success. I rise stronger after every setback, fortified by my resilience."

4. Gratitude for the Present:

Quote: "The more you praise and celebrate your life, the more there is in life to celebrate." – Oprah Winfrey

Affirmation: "I cherish each moment as a gift. My life is a celebration of the beautiful journey I've undertaken."

5. Wisdom of Aging:

Quote: "Aging is not 'lost youth,' but a new stage of opportunity and strength." – Betty Friedan

Affirmation: "With each passing year, I gain wisdom and resilience. I embrace the opportunities that come with age."

Setting Realistic Goals

1. Health-Focused Goals:

Goal: Engage in chair yoga sessions for at least 20 minutes three times a week.

Rationale: Gradually integrating physical activity contributes to enhanced flexibility and overall well-being.

2. Nutritional Objectives:

Goal: Incorporate one new nutrient-rich food item into meals each week.

Rationale: Building a diverse, nutrient-packed diet supports overall health and facilitates weight management.

3. Cognitive Wellness:

Goal: Dedicate 10 minutes a day to mental exercises such as puzzles or brain games.

Rationale: Regular mental stimulation is crucial for cognitive health and can be an enjoyable daily routine.

4. Social Engagement:

Goal: Attend a local seniors' group or virtual meetup at least once a month.

Rationale: Building social connections enhances emotional well-being and provides a sense of community.

5. Sleep Improvement:

Goal: Establish a consistent bedtime routine and aim for 7-8 hours of sleep each night.

Rationale: Quality sleep contributes to overall health, energy levels, and mood.

Building a Supportive Community
1. Local Seniors' Groups:

Initiative: Join local seniors' groups or community centres that offer diverse activities.

Benefit: Provides an opportunity to connect with peers, share experiences, and engage in group activities.

2. Virtual Communities:

Initiative: Explore online forums or social media groups dedicated to senior well-being.

Benefit: Connects seniors with a broader community, fostering shared interests and providing a platform for support.

3. Family and Friends Involvement:

Initiative: Share health goals with family and friends, encouraging their involvement.

Benefit: Builds a strong support system, with loved ones providing encouragement, motivation, and participation in activities.

4. Group Exercise Classes:

Initiative: Participate in local or virtual group exercise classes.

Benefit: Creates a sense of camaraderie, with shared fitness goals and the opportunity to encourage one another.

5. Mentorship Programs:

Initiative: Engage in mentorship programs where seniors can share experiences and advice.

Benefit: Fosters a supportive environment, offering guidance and companionship through shared life experiences.

Motivation for seniors extends beyond physical health goals; it's a holistic approach encompassing mental, emotional, and social well-being. Encouraging quotes and affirmations provide daily inspiration, realistic goals ensure progress, and building a supportive community offers a network of strength and camaraderie. By integrating these motivational tips, seniors can embark on a journey toward holistic well-being, embracing each day with resilience, purpose, and joy.

VI

Overcoming Challenges

Embarking on a wellness journey often comes with its own set of challenges, particularly for seniors. This section delves into overcoming obstacles with a specific focus on dealing with physical limitations, addressing potential health concerns, and the importance of modifying exercises to suit individual needs.

Dealing with Physical Limitations

1. Recognizing Personal Boundaries:

Effectively engaging in chair yoga with physical limitations begins with acknowledging and understanding individual boundaries. Embracing a mindset that values progress over perfection encourages seniors to establish a positive connection with their bodies, fostering self-compassion as they embark on their wellness journey.

2. Tailoring Chair Yoga Poses:

Collaborating with experienced chair yoga instructors becomes pivotal for tailoring poses to accommodate specific physical limitations.

Whether addressing mobility issues, joint stiffness, or discomfort, modifications can be applied to ensure a secure and effective practice. These personalized adjustments empower seniors to participate confidently, adapting poses to suit their comfort and requirements.

3. Gradual Advancement:

Implementing a gradual progression strategy is essential for adapting to new movements and minimizing strain. Commencing with simpler poses allows seniors to build confidence, gradually introducing more challenging postures as flexibility and strength improve. This methodical approach respects the body's natural pace, fostering a sense of achievement throughout the wellness journey.

4. Integration of Adaptive Tools:

Exploring the utilization of adaptive tools further enhances support during chair yoga sessions. Items like cushions, blocks, or resistance bands can be strategically introduced to provide additional stability and comfort. Adapting the environment to individual needs ensures a secure practice, promoting a positive and inclusive experience for seniors with diverse physical abilities.

5. Cultivating Patience and Tenacity:

Cultivating patience and tenacity becomes paramount when navigating chair yoga with physical limitations. Seniors are encouraged to celebrate small victories and focus on positive changes experienced along the way. Recognizing that progress may unfold gradually, each step forward becomes a testament to resilience and commitment, contributing to an overall sense of well-being.

6. Mindful Body Awareness:

Encouraging mindful self-awareness during chair yoga fosters a deeper connection with one's body. Seniors are prompted to attentively listen to their bodies, paying heed to sensations and adjusting movements accordingly. This heightened awareness empowers individuals to make informed decisions about their practice, creating a harmonious and mindful engagement with chair yoga.

7.Engaging in a Supportive Community:

Participating in a supportive community of fellow participants and understanding instructors plays a significant role in navigating physical limitations. The exchange of experiences, sharing of tips, and mutual encouragement cultivates camaraderie. This supportive environment not only boosts motivation but also provides a space for shared understanding as individuals navigate their distinct wellness paths.

Navigating physical limitations in chair yoga entails a comprehensive approach that includes recognizing personal boundaries, customizing poses, adopting gradual progression, integrating adaptive tools, fostering patience, promoting mindful body awareness, and engaging with a supportive community. By incorporating these elements, seniors can confidently embrace chair yoga, honouring their unique needs, celebrating progress, and cultivating an enriched sense of well-being.

Managing Potential Health Concerns

1. Thorough Medical Consultation:

Giving priority to a thorough medical consultation before commencing a chair yoga program is crucial, particularly for seniors with potential health concerns. Seeking advice from healthcare professionals ensures that exercise routines align with individual health conditions. This collaborative approach establishes a secure and customized foundation for the wellness journey.

2. Holistic Approach to Well-Being:

Encouraging a holistic approach to well-being involves addressing not only physical concerns but also mental and emotional facets. Seniors are encouraged to adopt practices that encompass stress management, quality sleep, and a balanced diet. This comprehensive strategy contributes to enhancing overall health, laying the groundwork for a more resilient and robust lifestyle.

3. Medication Awareness:

Maintaining awareness of medication side effects and interactions is pivotal for individuals with potential health concerns. Regular communication with healthcare providers ensures a seamless integration of wellness practices with existing medications. This heightened awareness facilitates informed decision-making and cultivates a health-conscious mindset during chair yoga sessions.

4. Adaptive Yoga for Specific Conditions:

Exploring adaptive yoga practices tailored for specific health conditions becomes integral in addressing potential concerns. Whether managing arthritis, osteoporosis, or cardiovascular issues, participating in classes led by instructors trained in adaptive techniques ensures that exercises are not only safe but also beneficial for specific health needs.

5. Mindful Self-Monitoring:

Embracing mindful self-monitoring practices during chair yoga sessions empowers seniors to detect early signs of discomfort or health concerns. Regularly checking in with one's body and emotions ensures a proactive approach to well-being. This mindful self-awareness enables individuals to make informed decisions about their practice, fostering a health-conscious and attentive engagement.

6. Emotional and Mental Well-Being:

Acknowledging the interconnectedness of emotional and mental well-being with physical health is essential. Seniors are encouraged to prioritize activities that contribute to positive mental states, such as relaxation techniques, mindfulness, and engaging in activities that bring joy. This holistic approach cultivates a resilient mindset and supports overall well-being.

7. Supportive Healthcare Network:

Establishing and maintaining a supportive healthcare network is instrumental in managing potential health concerns. Open communication with healthcare providers ensures that emerging issues are promptly addressed. This collaborative approach provides seniors with the confidence that their wellness journey is guided by a team of professionals invested in their health and safety.

Managing potential health concerns in chair yoga involves a proactive and comprehensive approach that includes a thorough medical consultation, embracing holistic well-being, medication awareness, adaptive practices for specific conditions, mindful self-monitoring, prioritizing emotional and mental well-being, and fostering a supportive healthcare network.

Customizing Exercises for Individuals
1. Tailored Fitness Plans:

Working collaboratively with fitness professionals allows the development of customized chair yoga plans tailored to individual needs and objectives. This personalized approach ensures exercises address specific challenges and support unique progress, fostering empowerment and inclusivity.

2. Varied Options for Diverse Fitness Levels:

Offering different variations for chair yoga poses accommodates a range of fitness levels within a group. Providing alternatives from novice to advanced levels enables everyone to engage at their own pace, creating a supportive and inclusive environment that encourages participation and advancement.

3. Personalized Progression:

Encouraging participants to advance at their own pace is crucial for effective exercise modification. Adapting routines based on personal comfort and capability promotes a sense of achievement and empowerment. This individualized approach contributes to a positive and sustainable chair yoga experience, encouraging adherence to the practice.

4. Responsive to Feedback and Adjustments:

Promoting open communication between participants and instructors invites feedback on exercise effectiveness and comfort. Regularly assessing and adjusting routines based on individual progress and feedback ensures that chair yoga remains tailored, relevant, and supportive of each participant's unique journey.

5. Cultivating an Inclusive Atmosphere:

Creating an inclusive environment emphasizes that modifications are a natural part of any fitness journey and do not diminish the value of one's efforts. Seniors are encouraged to embrace modifications without judgment, fostering a supportive atmosphere that celebrates diversity in abilities and ensures everyone can comfortably participate in chair yoga.

6. Mindful Adaptation for Injuries:

Addressing injuries or specific physical concerns requires a mindful adaptation of exercises. Instructors can collaborate closely with individuals to modify poses, incorporating alternatives that avoid strain on affected areas while still delivering the benefits of chair yoga. This personalized approach prioritizes safety and encourages participants to prioritize their well-being.

7. Tailoring Goals Individually:

Recognizing and respecting the unique goals of each participant is crucial in modifying exercises. Setting individualized fitness goals allows seniors to tailor their chair yoga practice to meet specific aspirations, whether it's enhanced flexibility, improved strength, or overall well-being. This personalized goal-setting fosters a sense of purpose and motivation.

In summary, customizing exercises for individuals in chair yoga involves developing tailored fitness plans, offering varied options for diverse fitness levels, promoting personalized progression, encouraging responsiveness to feedback and adjustments, cultivating an inclusive atmosphere, practicing mindful adaptation for injuries, and setting individualized goals. Embracing these practices ensures chair yoga remains adaptable and inclusive, catering to the diverse needs and goals of each participant for a positive and enriching experience.

VII

Celebrating Success

Embarking on a 90-day chair yoga weight loss plan is a commendable journey, and celebrating success is an integral part of fostering motivation and sustaining positive habits. This section delves into recognizing achievements along the way, reinforcing positive habits, and planning for continued well-being beyond the 90 days.

Acknowledging Milestones Along the Way

1. Setting Significant Milestones:

Establishing specific milestones throughout the 90-day chair yoga program provides participants with clear and achievable goals.

Celebrating the attainment of milestones, such as mastering challenging poses or consistently participating in sessions, acknowledges progress and inspires individuals to strive for subsequent achievements.

2. Encouraging Personal Reflections on Success:

Urging participants to maintain personal success journals enhances self-awareness and reflective practices.

Journaling about daily accomplishments, whether it's improved flexibility, reduced stress, or enhanced balance, reinforces the positive influence of chair yoga on overall well-being and cultivates a positive mindset.

3. Communal Celebrations:

Arranging regular group celebrations within the chair yoga community fosters a collective sense of achievement.

Commemorating shared accomplishments, whether through virtual gatherings or in-person events, nurtures camaraderie and strengthens the supportive community, motivating individuals to persist in their commitment to the program.

4. Presentation of Certificates of Achievement:

Recognizing participants with Certificates of Achievement at various intervals and upon completing the 90-day program serves as formal acknowledgment of their dedication and progress.

This concrete recognition becomes a source of pride, symbolizing their commitment to health and well-being, and serves as a visual reminder of their accomplishments.

5. Creation of Visual Progress Boards:

Developing visual progress boards where participants can visually track their achievements enhances motivation.

These boards may include personal goals, milestones, and visual representations of progress. Regularly updating and reflecting on these boards reinforces a sense of accomplishment and provides a visual testament to their journey.

6. Recognition on Social Media Platforms:

Encouraging participants to share their accomplishments on social media platforms offers a public avenue for acknowledgment.

Celebrating successes online not only acknowledges individual achievements but also inspires and motivates others within the community, creating a positive ripple effect.

7. Surprise Recognition Moments:

Incorporating unexpected recognition moments during chair yoga sessions adds an element of excitement and maintains participant engagement.

Randomly spotlighting individuals for their commitment, progress, or positive attitude reinforces the idea that every effort is valued and appreciated.

8.Peer Acknowledgment Sessions:

Integrating peer acknowledgment sessions provides participants with opportunities to recognize and celebrate each other's achievements.

Peer support and acknowledgment foster a positive atmosphere within the community, promoting a culture of encouragement and collective success.

9.Issuance of Personalized Achievement Badges:

Awarding personalized achievement badges for specific accomplishments introduces a fun and rewarding component to the journey.

These badges can range from consistent attendance to achieving particular fitness goals, providing participants with tangible symbols of their progress.

10.Facilitating Storytelling Sessions:

Hosting storytelling sessions where participants can share their success stories creates a source of inspiration.

Listening to the experiences of others reinforces the notion that each journey is unique, and every small step forward is deserving of celebration.

Incorporating these strategies for acknowledging achievements ensures participants feel recognized and motivated throughout their 90-day chair yoga weight loss plan. Celebrating success along the way becomes an integral and dynamic aspect of the wellness journey, encouraging sustained commitment and nurturing a positive mindset.

Strengthening Positive Habits

1. Continuous Application of Positive Reinforcement Techniques:

Employing consistent positive reinforcement techniques during chair yoga sessions establishes a nurturing environment.

Regularly acknowledging participants for their dedication, perseverance, and progress reinforces positive habits, cultivating a sense of accomplishment and ongoing motivation.

2. Structured Programs for Incentives:

Implementing structured incentive programs with rewards tied to specific milestones enhances motivational factors.

Recognizing achievements with incentives, whether they are wellness-oriented items or personalized experiences, strengthens the correlation between positive habits and tangible rewards.

3. Education on Habit Formation:

Providing informative resources on habit formation empowers participants to comprehend the science behind establishing positive routines.

Gaining insights into the cues, routines, and rewards integral to habit formation enables individuals to consciously shape their behaviour, ensuring the establishment of enduring positive habits.

4. Encouragement of Peer Accountability Partnerships:

Promoting the creation of peer accountability partnerships encourages mutual support.

Pairing individuals to check in on each other's progress, share challenges, and celebrate successes establishes a network that reinforces positive habits and instils a sense of responsibility.

5. Group Affirmations and Positive Reinforcement:

Integrating group affirmations and positive reinforcement during chair yoga sessions fosters a constructive and uplifting atmosphere.

Regularly expressing positive affirmations and offering encouraging words reinforces the understanding that positive habits contribute significantly to overall well-being, fostering a mindset aligned with healthy practices.

6. Acknowledgment of Consistency:

Recognizing and celebrating consistency in attendance and participation underscores the significance of forming regular positive habits.

Highlighting the commitment to the chair yoga program reinforces the belief that sustained engagement plays a crucial role in attaining wellness goals.

7. Interactive Workshops on Habit Formation:

Conducting interactive workshops cantered on habit formation equips participants with practical tools and strategies.

Sharing and learning effective techniques for integrating positive habits into daily life promotes a collective grasp of the impact of these habits on overall well-being.

8.Periodic Goal Setting and Review Sessions:

Facilitating sessions for periodic goal setting and reviews prompts participants to reflect on their progress.

Establishing new goals and revisiting existing ones ensures continued engagement and motivation, strengthening the positive habits established during the chair yoga program.

9.Engagement in Positive Habit Challenges:

Introducing challenges focused on positive habits within the chair yoga community encourages friendly competition and motivation.

Challenges may involve maintaining specific wellness routines, incorporating healthy practices, or adopting mindful habits, reinforcing positive behaviours through shared experiences.

10.Continuous Education on Healthy Practices:

Providing ongoing education on healthy practices beyond chair yoga sessions fortifies positive habits.

Participants benefit from learning about nutrition, stress management, and holistic well-being, further solidifying their commitment to a health-conscious lifestyle.

Incorporating these approaches to strengthen positive habits ensures that participants not only establish but also sustain healthy practices throughout and beyond the 90-day chair yoga weight loss plan. By fostering a supportive atmosphere, offering incentives, and fostering a shared understanding of habit formation, individuals are empowered to perpetuate positive habits for enduring well-being.

Strategizing for Sustained Well-being Post 90 Days

1. Adapting to Long-Term Routines:

Assisting participants in seamlessly transitioning from the structured 90-day plan to enduring wellness routines is crucial.

Highlighting the ongoing integration of chair yoga into daily life beyond the initial program ensures a sustained dedication to physical activity and holistic well-being.

2. Formulating Fresh Wellness Objectives:

Collaborating with participants to establish novel wellness goals post the initial 90 days sustains motivation.

Whether it encompasses mastering advanced yoga poses, exploring additional exercises, or targeting broader health goals, setting fresh objectives ensures sustained enthusiasm and a progressive approach to well-being.

3. Continuous Nutritional Guidance:

Providing continual nutritional guidance aids participants in upholding a balanced and healthful diet.

Educating on sustainable dietary habits ensures that the positive impact of chair yoga is complemented by nutritious choices, contributing to overall well-being extending beyond the structured program.

4. Extended Community Participation:

Encouraging ongoing involvement within the chair yoga community past the 90 days nurtures a lasting support network.

Facilitating regular events, workshops, or social gatherings keeps participants connected, reinforcing their dedication to well-being and supplying sustained encouragement.

5. Self-Reflection and Flexible Adaptation:

Empowering participants with tools for self-reflection allows them to adapt their routines based on evolving needs.

Regular contemplation of physical and emotional well-being enables informed choices, ensuring their wellness journey remains dynamic and adaptable to changing circumstances.

6. Mindful Integration of Holistic Practices:

Stressing the significance of mindfully incorporating various holistic practices into daily life promotes comprehensive well-being.

Encouraging the infusion of mindfulness, stress management techniques, and other positive habits ensures an inclusive approach to sustained mental and physical health.

7. Tailored Personal Well-being Plans:

Assisting participants in crafting personalized well-being plans tailored to their unique preferences and goals fosters autonomy.

Whether it involves a blend of chair yoga, outdoor activities, or mindfulness practices, customizing plans ensures individuals engage in activities they enjoy, fostering lasting adherence.

8. Educational Workshops on Long-Term Wellness:

Conducting informative workshops cantered on long-term wellness equips participants with knowledge for enduring health.

Topics may span stress management strategies, tips for maintaining a healthy lifestyle, and insights into the importance of ongoing self-care, delivering valuable tools for prolonged well-being.

9. Celebrating Achievements Beyond 90 Days:

Reinforcing the celebration of milestones and achievements even after the initial 90 days maintains a positive mindset.

Recognizing progress at regular intervals acts as a perpetual source of motivation, encouraging individuals to persist in their wellness journey.

10. Promoting Family and Social Support:

Emphasizing the role of family and social support in sustaining well-being motivates participants to involve their loved ones.

Cultivating a supportive environment at home and within social circles ensures individuals have a network that fortifies healthy habits, fostering an environment of enduring well-being.

In essence, devising strategies for sustained well-being post 90 days involves guiding participants in adapting to long-term routines, formulating new wellness objectives, providing continuous nutritional guidance, promoting extended community participation, encouraging self-reflection and flexible adaptation, mindfully integrating holistic practices, creating tailored well-being plans, organizing educational workshops, celebrating achievements, and fostering family and social support. By incorporating these components, individuals can smoothly integrate positive habits into their daily lives, ensuring a persistent commitment to their overall well-being.

Conclusion

Concluding this guide, let's revisit the extensive advantages chair yoga brings to seniors. From improved flexibility and balance to stress reduction and heightened mindfulness, chair yoga uniquely addresses the specific needs of seniors, fostering holistic well-being. Its gentle yet potent impact extends across physical, mental, and emotional dimensions.

Motivation for Ongoing Practice

As I bring this guide to a close, I want to express sincere encouragement for your continued engagement in chair yoga. The positive transformations witnessed during the 90-day weight loss plan are just the beginning. Consistency remains pivotal, and weaving chair yoga into your daily routine ensures an enduring journey towards improved health. Embrace the pleasure of movement, the calmness of mindful breathing, and the overall sense of well-being that chair yoga consistently delivers.

In concluding your ongoing wellness journey, remember that a network of support is readily accessible. Whether seeking additional chair yoga materials, nutritional insights, or a community of fellow enthusiasts, diverse resources await exploration. Here are final sentiments and resources to assist you:

Diversify Your Practices:

Consider exploring diverse chair yoga routines, targeting specific facets such as balance, strength, or relaxation. Variety ensures ongoing engagement and holistic benefits.

Nutritional Information:

Uphold a well-balanced diet for sustained well-being. Seek advice from nutritional sources or professionals to further refine your dietary choices in harmony with your fitness objectives.

Community Involvement:

Stay connected with the chair yoga community.
Attend local classes, participate in virtual
sessions, or engage in online forums to share
experiences, gain insights, and draw continuous
motivation.

Mindfulness Applications:

Infuse mindfulness into your daily routine with
meditation or mindfulness applications. These
tools offer guided sessions to foster mental
clarity and emotional equilibrium.

Utilize Fitness Tracking Tools:

Explore the use of fitness trackers to monitor your physical activity. Establishing daily goals and tracking progress can serve as a motivating factor in sustaining an active lifestyle.

Remember, your wellness journey is distinct, and your commitment to chair yoga is admirable. Continue embracing the benefits, maintain consistency, and celebrate the ongoing progress on your journey toward enhanced health and a more fulfilling life.

Suggested Resources for Ongoing Support:

- Online Chair Yoga Classes

- Nutritional Guidance Tailored for Seniors

- Mindfulness Meditation Apps

- Reviews on Fitness Tracking Devices

- Community Forums for Senior Well-being

In conclusion, may your path be marked by vigour, joy, and a profound sense of well-being. Here's to your ongoing journey toward a healthier and more joyful you!